Supernatural

Weight Loss

Heather O'Brien

Scripture quotations are taken from the Holy Bible, New Living Translation, copyright © 1996, 2004, 2007 by Tyndale House Foundation. Used by permission of Tyndale House Publishers, Inc., Carol Stream, IL 60188. All rights reserved.

International Standard Book Number:
978-1540357915 (Supernatural Weight Loss)

Photographs by *Jason O'Brien*

Printed in the United States of America

Second Printing 2021

Introduction

As I am sitting here eating my bowl of ice cream, I'm pondering the thought of supernatural weight loss. If I really died on the cross with Jesus, and He lives inside of me with all of His power and authority, why can't I pray this weight off of my body? The natural response is to reject that idea because it wouldn't involve me working for it. It is biblical to take care of the physical body as it is a temple of the Holy Spirit. Still, I yearn to know why it would be impossible since Jesus mentioned I could move a mountain if I had enough faith. I clearly have a mountain on my torso that I would like to "move" off of my body, so I'm pondering this thought of supernatural weight loss a bit more.

This thought process began a few years ago. I began to pray and seek the Lord about the idea of supernatural weight loss. I never felt that Jesus thought it was a stupid idea, so I continued to pray about it with Him. It wasn't long before I would try random prayers over my body just to see what would happen. The first prayer led to me losing 5 pounds overnight. It was a success! This small success led me to pray more and seek further success. Why only 5 pounds? Because He wanted me to seek out the mystery to be able to tell the world about supernatural weight loss. If it had happened over night, I would not have had the burning desire nor ability to proclaim to the world how to make it happen.

Proverbs 25:2 - It is the glory of God to conceal a matter; to search out a matter is the glory of kings.

We yearn to have a body that will allow us to enjoy food and dispose of the waste instead of holding tight to the extra pounds. Surely our supernatural body could supernaturally stay the right size. We are supernatural beings. Due to Jesus dying on the cross, and us accepting Him as our savior, He has given us access to all authority and power. We have been commissioned to heal the sick and raise the dead. If we have that kind of resurrection power with Jesus inside of us, nothing is impossible!

With this line of thinking, I began to practice some powerful prayers. While getting ready for work one morning, I went into my closet to get dressed. I remembered how the clothing did not wear out for 40 years while the Israelites were in the wilderness. If they wore the same clothes for 40 years, I cannot imagine that they would have a wardrobe full of varying sizes. So, if God could supernaturally keep their clothing from wearing out, it would not be a far stretch to just imagine that they possibly did not have weight gain/loss issues. So, while standing in my closet deciding what to wear, I prayed, "God, I believe that you could adjust my body to fit into these pants." So, I took a step of faith and put on a pair that would normally not fit me. They would not go up past my knees. I had a good giggle from that. So, I thought about that story in the Bible where the king only struck the ground 3 times and realized it was a test after he failed. So, I took another pair out and said, "I still have faith, Lord!" They did not fit either. So, I said, "Ok, maybe the third time will work," and I tried on another pair of pants. They did not fit either. I was about to be late to work doing all this so I just grabbed a pair of leggings and a dress and said, "God, I'll try again if that's what you want. I still believe."

A few months later, I did something even more outrageous. I wore a pair of pants to work that were so tight I could barely breathe. By wearing these extremely tight pants, I thought I was showing my faith that I believed God would fix my body by the time I got to work. I assumed this great faith would work, and I would not have to wear them all day in public. This act of faith did not make me smaller or my pants bigger. I just had to wear them unbuttoned all day.

Another time, I got a measuring tape out and prayed. I wrapped the measuring tape around my waist and told the fat to dissolve and the skin to shrink. Each time I prayed, the reading on the tape was smaller! It went down an inch through this process! But, it stopped moving after the inch. The fact that it moved was proof to me that I needed to keep searching out the possibility of supernatural weight loss.

During this process, I learned some vital information to the heart of my questions. Although I was seeking physical appearance changes, God wanted to make some internal changes. **These internal changes would create an environment within me that could sustain the physical changes when my prayer for supernatural weight loss was answered.** When the process seemed slow, I believed that it was only because the response would be greater than what I asked for initially.

Zechariah 4:10 - Do not despise these small beginnings, for the LORD rejoices to see the work begin, to see the plumb line in Zerubbabel's hand.

The phrase "and suddenly" in the Bible almost always is AFTER a process. For example, the Holy Spirit "suddenly fell upon them" after 10 days of prayer.

Chapter 1

Forgiveness For Others & Ourselves

In this book, I will be discussing many possible hindrances to you receiving supernatural weight loss. In each section, there will be a time for reflection on what is discussed and prayer examples. As forgiveness is an important part of living a Christian life, I'm first going to take time to discuss a three step model.

Forgiveness is a threefold process. First, we must confess our sins, including bitter roots towards others and ourselves. **<u>Ask forgiveness</u>** for these sins in a very specific manner. You would not let your child get away with simply saying, "I am sorry." Rather, you would ask your child to specify what they were sorry for in detail. Second, we must **<u>release all judgments</u>**. Judging yourself or others is a sin. It is equally important to release those who have judged you. Third, we must be able to **<u>bless</u>** those who have hurt us. The process of forgiveness is not complete until you can wholeheartedly bless the offender (even if it is yourself).

Forgiveness does not mean you have to be best friends with the person who hurt you. It simply means you have given the situation over to God to handle. If you have difficulty with this process, remember how much Jesus has forgiven you. Jesus loves you just as much as He loves the person who hurt you.

Bitterness and envy are not fruit from the Holy Spirit. When we compare ourselves to others, we inevitably rob ourselves of our own joy. Sometimes, we jokingly bad mouth others who are thinner and more in shape than us, but it is not a fruit of the Spirit. Bitterness and envy are helping to store on your extra pounds. This is called the law of sowing and reaping. Judgments are not for humans. All judgment is for Jesus and only for one particular day...the Judgment Day. Keep that in mind the next time you see someone with a fit body. Decide to speak life over them instead of negative words. There is power of life and death in the tongue.

When you can speak love towards others who prosper and are in good health, you will find yourself in a position to receive the same rewards they have received.

Forgiveness: 3-Step Process

Forgive. Release. Bless.

Forgive: Forgive Offenders, Yourself, and/or God (per offense and be specific).

Matt 18:34-35 -Then the angry king sent the man to prison to be tortured until he had paid his entire debt. "That's what my

heavenly Father will do to you if you refuse to forgive your
*brothers and sisters from your **heart**."*

Release Judgments: Where there is rotten fruit in our lives, there are rotten roots at the source. There are four types of judgments mentioned in the scripture that I have uncovered. These judgments keep us tied to the very thing we want separation from in life. As we walk by the Spirit, we will feel convictions at times to forgive others or ourselves. When we fail to follow this prompting, we allow unforgiveness to fester, creating roots of bitterness.

*Hebrews 12:14-15 - Work at living in peace with everyone, and work at living a holy life, for those who are not holy will not see the Lord. Look after each other so that none of you fails to receive the grace of God. Watch out that no poisonous **root of bitterness** grows up to trouble you, corrupting many.*

1. Law of honoring mother & father:
   Deuteronomy 5:16 - "Honor your father and mother, as the LORD your God commanded you. Then you will live a long, full life in the land the LORD your God is giving you.

2. Law of judging/receiving others:
   Matthew 7:1-2 - "Do not judge others, and you will not be judged. For you will be treated as you treat others. The

standard you use in judging is the standard by which you will be judged.

3. <u>Law of sowing & reaping:</u>
   Galatians 6:7 - Don't be misled--you cannot mock the justice of God. You will always harvest what you plant.

4. <u>Law of becoming what we judge:</u>
   Romans 2:1 - You may think you can condemn such people, but you are just as bad, and you have no excuse! When you say they are wicked and should be punished, you are condemning yourself, for you who judge others do these very same things.

<u>Bless:</u> Ask God to bless the person who has offended you. If you can do this AND mean it, you have thoroughly forgiven from your <u>heart</u>. When you recall the past hurtful situation, the memory may still be intact, but the pain associated with the memory will be wiped away once you have completely forgiven, released, and blessed the offender.

Prayer Time:

When you have some alone time, pray this simple prayer out loud. This prayer needs to be prayed before you continue your journey to supernatural weight-loss so there are no hindrances.

> *Father God, please show me if there is anyone I need to forgive. I ask that you would give me your grace and empower me to forgive them.*

> *Father God, please show me if there are any judgments I am holding towards anyone. I ask that you would give me your grace and empower me to release them.*

If God showed you anything during these prayers, take time to talk to Him fully about these matters. Follow the 3-step forgiveness prayer model of forgive, release, and bless for each offense.

Chapter 2

Love

The process of becoming skinny starts with your thoughts. Creating positive thinking about yourself is a process of consciously recognizing what we think and say about ourselves and readjusting those statements to be positive. Negative words over yourself keep your extra pounds locked in and pushed on tight. One of the first things I felt God wanted me to do was to start watching how I spoke about myself. I realized it was easy for me to put myself down and to think negatively about my looks. Once I recognized the negativity, I began replacing my thoughts and words. I began rewording simple phrases. For instance, instead of saying, "I'm fat" I began saying, "I have a few extra pounds on my body that I can get off easily." The more I changed these negative words and thoughts, the more it became what I believed.

I also started a regimen of looking in the mirror daily and saying, "You are beautiful!" out loud. I would say this every time I would see myself in a reflection throughout the day. The intention was to remind myself, and I would eventually believe and become this truth. After months of this process, I felt God ask me, "Why is it so hard to believe this truth that you are beautiful? It shouldn't be so much work to see the truth." These simple negative "beliefs" were strongholds in my life that needed to be driven out!

2 Corinthians 10:5 We demolish arguments and every pretension that sets itself up against the knowledge of God, and we take captive every thought to make it obedient to Christ.

I do believe there was a generational stronghold passed down to me. A stronghold is a thinking pattern based on lies and faulty belief systems. Strongholds cause us to believe lies that are against God's desires. **The most common lies are having incorrect images in our mind of who God is, how He sees us, and how we see ourselves.**

Strongholds are birthed and dwell in deception. The natural cure is to bring truth from God's Word to refute the lies. The more truth that can be brought to the lie, the more darkness must flee. Jesus tells us that we can be held in bondage due to strongholds in our lives. And His solution was to abide in His word.

John 8:32 And you will know the truth, and the truth will set you free.

Strongholds are torn down as God's Word is meditated on and soaked in. As the truth from the Word gets into your mind, it will eventually get into your heart. If you struggle realizing how much God loves you, spend time learning what God did to give His son Jesus to die for you. The price Jesus paid was for the joy set before HIm to see you living life fully and in abundance. The "truth" was that I was made in God's image. I didn't make myself, and I had no right to speak nor think negatively about myself.

Another lie that many believe is there is a genetic curse causing them to be fat. This is a lie that I believed too. Jesus died as THE curse. I refuse to believe this lie that genetics are to blame any longer. I canceled that genetic curse all the way back to Adam and all the way until Jesus comes again and you can also. Just simply believe Jesus did all He said He did for you.

After all of the lies have received truth, the most vital truth you must receive is how much you are loved. Love is one of the most important components to thinking yourself skinny. To love oneself is vital. If you cannot love yourself, you cannot give love or receive it from others easily.

You must be able to see yourself as beautiful when you are overweight and when you are the weight you want to be. When you are able to love yourself unconditionally, you will be spiritually healthy no matter what your weight is. Pour love into yourself in whatever manner that looks like to you. It is important to see yourself as God sees you. He made us in His image and He said it was good. If God says it is good, then it is not ok to argue with Him.

If you feel like your eating habits represent more of an addiction or if you suffer from other addictive behaviors, learning who you are in Christ and how much God loves you is the first step towards losing that bondage. The only way to truly overcome self-worth issues is to change how you see yourself in light of how God sees and loves you. To receive lasting freedom and wholeness, you will need to deal with any issues that have caused you to limit your capacity to receive all that God has for you.

Prayer Time:

When you have some alone time, pray this simple prayer out loud. After praying each sentence, close your eyes and wait for the Holy Spirit to reveal to you the answers to the prayer.

> *Holy Spirit, I ask that you reveal to me every dark thought I have about myself. Show me where this thought originated.*

Say this prayer for each dark thought and wait patiently while the Holy Spirit shows you the origination of each. After you are shown the origin of the bad thought about yourself, follow the 3-step process of forgiveness for yourself. Ask forgiveness to God for thinking badly of yourself, release judgments, and bless your body.

Now, conclude this prayer:

> *Please show me what you think about me. Now, I pray that my thoughts will be just like your thoughts for I have the mind of Christ (1 Cor 2:16).*

Chapter 3

Comfort

Where does your comfort come from? When you have a rough day or week, where do you turn for relief and comfort? Do you watch TV endlessly to get your mind off of the current issues? Do you have a glass or two of wine to ease the pain? Do you have food in your mouth to comfort you? The Holy Spirit wants to be your comforter. If you look to anything besides Him to comfort you, you are looking in the wrong place. Your pain and burdens will not get healed and lifted until you lean towards the Holy Spirit. He wants to be your only source of relief.

If you are seeking avenues to keep you busy instead of facing underlying pain, you are only covering it up. The way to end pain is to face it. Identify the source of your pain. Go all the way back to the first time you experienced this pain. Face it head-on with Jesus. He will not take you there to bring about more pain. He will bring you to that experience so that He can bring healing and restoration. Jesus actually bore our shame on the cross. If you are holding on to shame from your past, give it to Jesus. In exchange for your shame He would like to give you a double portion of honor. If you are hiding something and walking in shame you will never 100% be authentic with relationships in your life. Tell shame to go and replace it with your true identity of a life full of joy and honor.

Isaiah 61:7 - Instead of shame and dishonor, you will enjoy a double share of honor. You will possess a double portion of prosperity in your land, and everlasting joy will be yours.

If you can think of a time or many times when you have reached for something other than the Holy Spirit for comfort, you need to ask forgiveness. Ask the Holy Spirit to be your only source of comfort. Ask Him to remind you of this the next time you are in need so that you will learn to always look to Him for comfort and relief. The Holy Spirit is called The Comforter because there will be uncomfortable times when you need Him to comfort you.

Prayer Time:

When you have some alone time, pray this simple prayer out loud and wait for the Holy Spirit to reveal to you the answers.

Jesus, please show me if there are any past painful experiences that I have not brought to you. Walk with me to bring healing to those areas of my life.

Tell me where you were when they happened.

Empower me to forgive anyone who caused this hurt.

Now, please show me what or who I have reached to for comfort instead of you.

After you are shown the answer to your question, follow the 3-step process of forgiveness. The prayer may look something like this:

I ask that you forgive me for reaching to (insert your source of comfort) when I was not feeling well. Please help me to remember to always reach to you, My Comforter, any time I am in need of comfort.

Chapter 4

Worship

Is knowledge power? Will understanding calories and nutrition labels really be the key to your success in losing the extra pounds for good? I learned a lot about nutrition after losing 100 pounds a few years ago. I learned all about calories and which foods were the best choices. I spent time and money with weight loss clubs learning this information. It seems wrong to throw that information out the window. It was a form of revelation from God to understand what was contained in the items I was eating. My most used phrase at the time was "knowledge is power" because I honestly never understood calories, fat, fiber, protein, etc. Once I did, it was like a veil was lifted that I never knew existed. The problem with all of this knowledge was that I thought about food constantly. With every waking thought I would wonder how much I can eat now and still eat later. My thoughts about food overwhelmed me, and I surely was not focused on God. So, is this a valid point that "knowledge is power" or is it just a facade that the devil used to make me think about nothing but food?

The knowledge and wisdom I gained about calories and nutritional content was from God. He is the only reason I was able to comprehend what I did. I cannot throw that out. Knowledge is power. But, power must be used with God, not left up to man. We must let the Spirit guide us in truth about nutrition, but we must not be a slave to nutritional labels and calorie counting. If we let calorie counting rule our thinking and we become obsessed with nutrition, it becomes our idol. The Holy Spirit wants us to lean on Him for all truth, knowledge, comfort, and power. He will lead us down the correct path for weight loss. If you veer too far one way, you will become obsessed with food and weight. If you veer too far the other way, you will cast off restraint and lose your vision for the skinny mold of the person you want to be. The path that is correct is narrow and can only be found by trusting in the Holy Spirit to lead you into all truth.

You can't delete God given desires. However, they are easily perverted if not managed by the power of the Holy Spirit. Wanting to eat is a God given desire. The way we choose to eat will determine if we are doing it in a Godly manner.

Worship is the most important action in the world because worship transforms you into what you are worshiping. If you worship the food you eat, then "you are what you eat."

Adam & Eve decided to lean on their own understanding when they were being tricked by the serpent in the garden. They didn't know their decision was actually deciding to worship the serpent instead of God. They were tricked by relying on their own understanding instead of asking God why they weren't allowed to eat that particular fruit.

The devil is out to pervert and twist all of our God given desires. If we eat out of rage, anxiety, loneliness, hurt, or any other emotion, we are perverting the God given desire to eat. There aren't specific rules for food any more as it is all permissible. But, there is a Godly way to eat, and it won't be found by our own human understanding.

Prayer Time:

When you have some alone time, pray this prayer if you have noticed you focus too much of your attention on anything other than God. Some examples would be nutrition labels, exercise, meals, etc. Allow the Holy Spirit to speak to you directly on this topic.

> *Father, please forgive me if I have put (insert your idols here) above knowing and loving you. I ask that you empower me to release these idols from my life. I want you to be the one I worship and adore.*

Chapter 5

Dieting

You cannot use a negative emotion to motivate you into something positive. The word "diet" has the word "die" in it. **You will not get skinny by hating being fat.** I think it is important to understand that we will have to restrain ourselves by using the Holy Spirit as our guide and comforter. We may have to restrain ourselves from eating milkshakes or doughnuts all day long. However, the Holy Spirit can even help with that! We do not have to do anything apart from Him!

1 Corinthians 6:12-20 - You say, "I am allowed to do anything"—but not everything is good for you. And even though "I am allowed to do anything," I must not become a slave to anything. You say, "Food was made for the stomach, and the stomach for food." (This is true, though someday God will do away with both of them.) Don't you realize that your bodies are actually parts of Christ? Don't you realize that your body is the temple of the Holy Spirit, who lives in you and was given to you by God? You do not belong to yourself, for God bought you with a high price. So you must honor God with your body.

Still, when I contemplate dieting, I do not get excited. I actually think of reasons why I should not do it. I am reminded of a pair of running shoes that I got in middle school. These shoes were my one nice pair that I got for the school year. They were name-brand and looked really nice. I got home and wore them around the house. They seemed perfect, so I wore them to school the next day. By the end of the day, my feet were sore. There was some hard plastic on the sides that poked into my feet leaving sores. So, the next day, I loosened the shoe strings. I thought that making them looser would definitely keep them from hurting my feet. But, my feet could not stay in the shoes with them that loose, and the hard plastic was still poking my feet. I tried to wear these shoes at least once a week hoping that I could wear them into use. I could not take them back to the store since I had already worn them around outside. They were expensive and name-brand! They should be like fluffy clouds on my feet by now! However, I felt like I was wearing thorns inside of my socks. After months of trying to force them to not hurt, I finally gave up the battle.

Similarly, we try to diet to lose weight. We adjust our eating habits. We record everything that goes into our mouths. We pursue weight-loss sometimes at high prices and with pills that may kill us. The dieting never ends though. It becomes a lifelong event of loving and hating food. As hard as we work at eating less or eating the "right" foods, we still struggle to get to the weight we would truly like to be. Our struggles seem like never ending failures. We give up sometimes and restart in a month or a year. Either way, we always find the same results.

The problem with dieting, besides the dying part, is that we are using our own manpower to fuel the process. We have possibly envisioned a model-shaped body we want to attain and that is our primary focus of achievement. I'd like to propose that God has a perfect version of our body He intended for each of us to have. With His vision in front of us, His Spirit guiding us, and with His grace empowering us, we will have everything we need to achieve the body we were intended to have.

Proverbs 29:18 - Where there is no prophetic vision, the people cast off restraint. But happy is he who keeps the law.

Vision gives pain a purpose. Sometimes there are aches and pains when we need to adjust our lifestyles. Whether we need to quit eating ice cream before bed, take a walk a few times a week, or quit watching so much television, the "pain" of the change is usually well worth the results. It is important to be able to view yourself as the size you want to be. This "prophetic vision" gives you hope. To hope towards a future event is to inject power in your faith.

Prayer Time:

When you have some alone time, close your eyes and ask God to show you how He sees you.

Ask Him for a vision of what the perfect you looks like.

Ask Him what His perfect model of you looked like when He first knew you.

Let this vision be the only vision you keep about your desired looks. Do not look to society's ideals of perfection for your body.

Chapter 6

New Beginnings

You will never be able to let anyone love you more than you love you. The best way to accomplish that is to realize that you were made in the image of God. You look just like Him and His spirit lives within you. Don't compare yourself to anyone but God. You can love yourself because He first loved you. He knew what He was getting into when He made you, and He said it was "good." You are good. You are kind. You are merciful. You are beautiful and altogether lovely. You are God's child. That's why you can love you. And it's the only reason you should love you. Your love for yourself can't ever be based in your current season of life, how your clothes fit, or what kind of friends you have. You love you because God loves you. God was the painter, Jesus was the model, and you are the painting.

I have written this book as if you were a child of God. Whether you have given your life to Jesus or not, you are God's child. If you want to receive all the benefits of being His child, and you haven't asked Jesus to be your savior, it is time now. Simply ask Jesus to forgive you of your sins, and confess that He is now and forever Lord of your life. Start following Jesus by surrounding yourself with other believers, reading the Bible, and worshiping. You will be transformed as you draw near to Him.

Now, I will say a prayer for you and I believe that as you read this, the Holy Spirit will breathe new life into you and you will be transformed inside and out:

Father, thank you for the readers of this book. I ask that you would bless them with revelation knowledge on how to receive your love, how to love themselves, and how to love others as you intended. I speak love into their body, soul, and spirit right now. I pray the power of the Holy Spirit would come upon them and they would feel the fire of God burning within them. I ask that you would burn away any impurities and leave the precious gold you intended.

Father, if it is their heart's desire to lose fat, I ask that you would send your Holy Spirit to their bodies right now. Let the fat be a sweet burning sacrifice before you. Body, create muscle to burn the fat. Skin, tighten as the fat melts away. Any excess fat, it is time to go right now in the name of Jesus. Body shrink down to the size God intended for this body.

Father, I ask that you would do this amazing work within each person who desires such changes. I believe Jesus died for so many things including this precious prayer request to lose weight and excess fat. Jesus has already paid the price. Let today's supernatural weight-loss be just one of the joys that was set before Jesus to endure that horrible cross where He died for us.

Amen.

Follow the author for more resources and ideas:

Website: https://heatherobrien.net

Facebook: @MotherOfMillions

Facebook: @theblissteam

Instagram: @heather.w.obrien

Podcast: The Power of Four

Email: heather.w.obrien@outlook.com

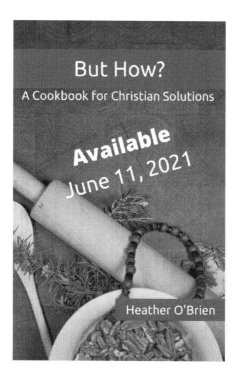

But How?
A Cookbook for Christian Solutions

Available
June 11, 2021

Heather O'Brien

This book offers recipes for greater success as a Christian and can lead to improved health physically, mentally, and spiritually. Each recipe was developed from personal questions, struggles, or desires for breakthrough.

Potential benefits:
- addictions ending
- emotions controlled
- understanding how to use and receive the gifts of healing and speaking in tongues
- learning how to forgive, hear God's voice, and steward the mundane

Made in the USA
Columbia, SC
29 January 2024

30486814R10026